Contents

Gastric sleeve surgery
Gastric Sleeve Diet: Everything You Need To Know To Lose Weight and Live better with the Vertical Sleeve. A Step By Step Guide For Planning What to Do and Eat Before and After Your Surgery

Alex Martinez
Introduction

Gastric Sleeve Surgery is now the hottest weight reduction operation on earth and causes significant and rapid weight reduction. Laparoscopic Sleeve Gastrectomy also referred to as the sleeve entails removing roughly 80 percent of their gut. The rest of the stomach is really a tubular pouch which looks like a banana. Gastric Sleeve surgery may be suitable weight reduction treatment for patients that aren't qualified for additional surgical procedures because of risk factors associated with a high BMI or other health conditions, including nausea. By abiding by the post-operative recommendations patients may expect to lose about 1 kilogram a week till their entire body weight reaches a healthful range. Because of a decrease in ghrelin, a hormone which affects appetite, patients will also be less inclined to feel hungry between meals. Restricts the total amount of food the stomach can hold - that the new stomach pouch carries a much smaller quantity than the standard gut and helps to significantly lower the total amount of food (and therefore calories) which may be consumed. The increased effect, but seems like the impact the surgery has on bowel tissues such as Ghrelin, the appetite hormone, which favourably suppresses appetite, reduces hunger, enhances satiety and enhances blood glucose control.gastric Sleeve surgery has a range of benefits over other weight loss processes. These are: Digestion works are preserved since the sole change is made to the dimensions of their gut.

Stomach nerves and openings remain intact and unaltered. The process for Gastric Sleeve surgery is laparoscopic, instead of open, meaning it's not as invasive, scarring will be minimal, and restoration will be faster.

As Gastric Sleeve surgery doesn't affect the digestive tract, healing times are somewhat faster than in other processes. Lower prospect of complications such as ulcers and other dangers related to gastric bypasses and lap-band surgeries. Involves a relatively short hospital stay of about 2 days When you have type 2 diabetes, evidence indicates that this ought to be a lot easier to control.

The disadvantages of Sleeve Gastrectomy will be the prospect of long term vitamin deficiencies, but this may be addressed by diet.

Chapter 1 what is gastric sleeve how it works?

CENTER FOR METABOLIC AND WEIGHT LOSS SURGERY

Sleeve gastrectomy is a surgical process that induces Weight loss by restricting food consumption. During this process, which is normally done laparoscopically, the surgeon removes about 75 percent of their gut. This ends in the gut taking on the form of a tube or "sleeve" that retains much less food. Although originally invented as the very first phase of a two phase process of superobese or high-risk sufferers, the sleeve gastrectomy is currently commonly and successfully used as a destination process for weight loss in men with BMI over 40.

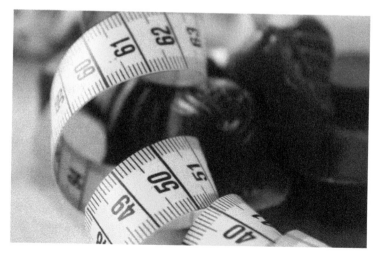

Gastric Sleeve

Statistically the documented weight loss with this particular process Ranges from 60 percent of their extra fat; better results are obtained with great adherence to dietary and behaviorial guidelines. With intelligent food choices, regular exercise and decent eating habits, individuals who've experienced a sleeve gastrectomy will appreciate and preserve decent weight reduction.

Together with the sleeve gastrectomy there's no foreign body Implanted, much like all the adjustable gastric band, and there's not any intricate intestinal rearrangement, much like all the gastric bypass. Many patients find that following a fair recovery, they are ready to comfortably eat a huge array of foods, such as meats and fibrous veggies. Contrary to the adjustable gastric band as well as also the gastric bypass, the sleeve gastrectomy is a permanent procedure -- it can't be reversed.

Removing some of the gut reduces the body's degree Of a hormone called ghrelin, which is often known as the "hunger hormone" Thus, a lot of men and women discover they are not as hungry following the sleeve gastrectomy. Ghrelin also plays a part in blood glucose metabolism, so individuals with type II diabetes often find an immediate decline in their need for diabetes drugs (particularly oral drugs) following the sleeve gastrectomy.

Advantages of Sleeve Gastrectomy

Sleeve gastrectomy induces rapid and effective weight loss much like gastric bypass surgery. Patients may expect to lose 50 percent or more of the extra weight in 3 years. The process doesn't require implantation of a ring, nor does this re-route the digestive procedure. Hormonal changes following the process assist patients to feel fuller eat, in addition to improve or solve diabetes.

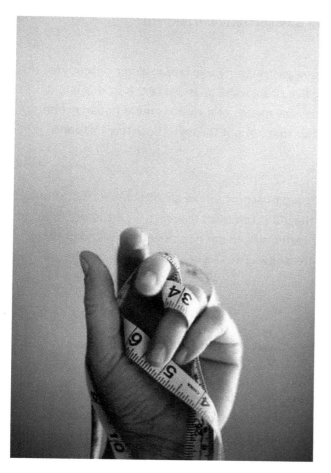

Disadvantages of Sleeve Gastrectomy

Like other surgical procedures, sleeve gastrectomy is non-reversible. The speed of premature surgical complications is similar to conventional gastric bypass. Patients are at risk for long term nutrient deficiencies.

What's Sleeve Gastrectomy Performed?

We do the sleeve gastrectomy as a laparoscopic procedure. This entails making five or six small incisions in the stomach and doing the process by means of a video camera (laparoscope) and lengthy tools that are put through these tiny incisions.

Throughout the laparoscopic sleeve gastrectomy (LSG), about 75 percent of the gut is removed leaving a lean gastric "tube" or "sleeve". No intestines have been removed or spilled through the sleeve gastrectomy. The LSG requires one or two hours to finish.

How Can Sleeve Gastrectomy Cause Weight Loss?

Sleeve gastrectomy is a restrictive process. It greatly reduces the size of your belly and restricts the total amount of food which may be consumed at any time. It doesn't cause decreased absorption of nourishment or bypass the own intestines. After eating a little bit of food, you'll feel full very fast and continue to feel full for many hours.

Sleeve gastrectomy can also lead to a reduction in appetite. In Addition to reducing the size of their gut, sleeve gastrectomy can lessen the sum of "hunger hormone" produced by the gut that might bring about weight loss following this process.

Who Would We Provide Laparoscopic Sleeve Gastrectomy?

This process is primarily used as part of a staged Strategy to surgical weight reduction. Patients that have a rather large body mass index (BMI) or who are at risk for undergoing a lengthier process because of lung or heart problems may benefit from the staged approach. Sometimes the choice to move ahead with a two-stage strategy is created before surgery because of such known risk factors. Quite simply, the choice to do sleeve gastrectomy (rather than gastric bypass) is created throughout the surgery. Reasons for creating this choice intraoperatively incorporate an overly big liver or scar tissue which would cause the gastric bypass process overly long or harmful.

In patients who experience LSG as a primary phase process, the Second phase (gastric bypass) is done 12 to 18 months after after substantial weight loss has happened and the possibility of anesthesia is a lot lower (and also the liver has diminished in size). Though this strategy involves two procedures, we think it's effective and safe for patients.

Laparoscopic sleeve gastrectomy may also be utilized as a Principal procedure. There's relatively little information concerning the use of LSG as a standalone process in patients with lower BMI's and it ought to be regarded as an investigational process in this patient category.

What Are The Dangers of Laparoscopic Sleeve Gastrectomy?

There are dangers that are typical to any laparoscopic Process like bleeding, infection, injury to other organs, or the requirement to convert to an open process. There's also a small risk of a flow from the basic line used to split the gut. These issues are infrequent and significant complications occur less than 1 percent of their time.

Overall, the operative risks associated with LSG are slightly greater than those found using the laparoscopic adjustable group but lower compared to the dangers related to gastric bypass.

What Are The Advantages Of Laparoscopic Sleeve Gastrectomy?

Based on their pre-operative weight, patients may expect to drop between 40% to 70 percent of the excess body fat in the first year following surgery.

Much obesity-related comorbidity improves or fix after bariatric surgery. Diabetes, hypertension, obstructive sleep apnea and abnormal cholesterol levels have been treated or improved in over 75 percent of patients experiencing LSG. Though long-term studies aren't yet accessible, the weight loss that happens after LSG contributes to remarkable improvement in those medical conditions from the first year following surgery.

Is Laparoscopic Sleeve Gastrectomy A Great Choice For Me?

Your physician may speak with you about LSG instead if you Have a BMI over 60 or important medical issues that increase your risk for getting anesthesia or gastric bypass. Laparoscopic sleeve gastrectomy might also be provided as part of a clinical evaluation when you've got a lower BMI and diabetes.

You should discuss all the available surgical procedures Together with your physician and decide which process is ideal for you.

Things to Know About Gastric Sleeve Weight Loss Surgery

1 approach to tackle obesity would be with regular surgery. This Kind of surgery involves removing or diminishing the size of your tummy. Bariatric surgery typically contributes to rapid weight reduction.

Gastric sleeve surgery is one of several Kinds of bariatric Surgery choices. Medical professionals typically call it vertical sleeve gastrectomy.

In this Guide, you'll have a closer look at what is involved in gastric sleeve surgery, such as its efficacy and potential complications.

What exactly does gastric sleeve surgery demand?

Gastric sleeve surgery is almost always performed as a invasive procedure using a laparoscope. This usually means a very long, thin tube is inserted into your abdomen through several tiny incisions. This tube has a light and a small camera attached to it and many tools.

Gastric sleeve surgery is performed with general anesthesia, which is medication that puts you right into a really deep sleep and takes a ventilator to breathe for you during the surgery.

The surgery involves dividing your gut into 2 unequal Components. Approximately 80 percent of those outer curved portion of your gut is cut off and removed.

The advantages of the remaining 20 percent are then stapled or sutured together. This produces a banana-shaped stomach that is just about 25% of its initial size.

You are going to be at the living room about one hour. After the Surgery is finished, you're going to be moved into the recovery area for health care. You are going to be at the recovery area for one more hour or so as you awaken from the anesthesia.

The tiny incisions in your abdomen typically cure fast. The minimally invasive nature of this surgery makes it possible to recuperate faster than a process where your stomach is started using a bigger incision.

Unless there are complications, you should have the Ability to go Home within two or three days following the surgery.

Is it successful?

Gastric sleeve surgery helps you Eliminate weight in two manners:

• Your Stomach is considerably smaller in order to feel full and stop eating earlier. As a result, that you take in fewer calories.

• The component of the stomach that generates ghrelin -- a hormone that is connected with appetite -- has been eliminated, which means you are much less hungry.

According to the American Society of Metabolic and Allergic Surgery, you can expect to lose at least 50 per cent of your extra weight over the 18 to 24 weeks after gastric sleeve surgery. Some people today lose 60 to 70 percent .

It is Important to Keep in Mind that this Is Only Going to happen if you Are dedicated to adhering to the diet and exercise plan recommended by the physician. By embracing these lifestyle modifications, you are more inclined to keep the weight off long term.

Weight reduction benefits

Losing a significant Number of excess weights can improve Your quality of life also make it less difficult to carry out many daily tasks.

Another important advantage of weight reduction is that the reduced risk Of obesity-related wellness conditions. These include:

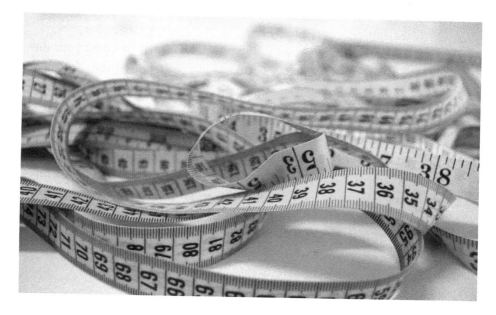

• Type 2 diabetes

• Significant cholesterol (hyperlipidemia)

• Significant Blood pressure (hypertension)

• Obstructive Sleep apnea

Who's a fantastic candidate for this surgery?

Bariatric surgery of any type, such as gastric sleeve Surgery, is just considered choice when powerful efforts to boost your diet and exercise habits, and also the usage of weight-loss drugs, have not worked.

Even after that, you have to meet specific standards to be eligible for a regular procedure. These standards are based on the own body mass index (BMI) and if you have some obesity-related wellness conditions.

Qualifying conditions:

• Intense (morbid) obesity (BMI rating of 40 or greater)

• Obesity (BMI rating of 35 to 39) with one important obesity-related condition

Sometimes, gastric sleeve surgery is completed if you are Obese but do not fulfill the standards for obesity, however, you get a substantial health condition associated with your weight.

What are the complications and risks?

Gastric sleeve surgery is known as a relatively safe procedure. But like all significant surgeries, there may be dangers and complications.

Some complications may happen after any surgery. All these include:

• Hemorrhage. Bleeding in your surgical wound or within your body may result in shock when it is intense.

• Deep vein thrombosis (DVT). Surgery as well as the healing procedure can boost your chance of a blood clot forming on your vein, usually in a leg vein.

• Pulmonary embolism. A pulmonary embolism can occur when a part of a blood clot breaks off and travels to your lungs.

• Irregular heartbeat. Surgery may boost the danger of an irregular pulse, particularly atrial fibrillation.

• Pneumonia. Pain can permit you to take shallow breaths that may result in a lung disease, such as pneumonia.

Gastric sleeve surgery may have added complications. A few possible side effects that are specific to this surgery include:

• Gastric leaks. Stomach fluids can flow in the suture line on your gut where it had been stitched back together.

• Stenosis. Section of your gastric sleeve may shut, resulting in an obstruction in your stomach.

• Vitamin deficiencies. The part of your gut that is eliminated is partially responsible for the absorption of vitamins that your body needs. If you don't take vitamin supplements, then this may result in deficiencies.

• Heartburn (GERD). Reshaping your gut can cause or aggravate heartburn. This may normally be treated with over-the-counter drugs.

It is Important to Keep in Mind that changing your diet and Exercise habits are crucial to losing the weight and keeping it off following gastric sleeve surgery. It is potential to gain the weight back if you

- eat also much

- consume an unhealthy diet

- exercise too little

Other concerns

Another Frequent concern, especially Once You Eliminate Lots of Weight fast, is that the massive number of surplus skin you might be left with as the pounds drop away. This is a frequent complication of gastric sleeve surgery.

This excess skin could be removed if it disturbs you. But remember it may take around 18 months for the body to stabilize following gastric sleeve surgery. That is why it's generally better to wait until considering a skin removal process. Until then, you might want to try out some strategies for tightening loose skin.

Another thing to think about before choosing to have gastric Sleeve surgery is that, unlike any other regular surgeries, gastric sleeve surgery is permanent. If you aren't satisfied with the outcome, your tummy cannot be transformed back to how it was.

How can your diet alter following gastric sleeve surgery?

Before gastric sleeve surgery is completed, you typically must consent to particular lifestyle modifications recommended by your physician. These changes are supposed to assist you reach and sustain weight loss.

One of these changes involves eating a healthy diet for the remainder of your life.

Your physician will recommend the very best gastric sleeve diet to get you after your surgery. The dietary modifications your surgeon proposes may be like the overall dietary guidelines under.

Dietary changes

• Two weeks Prior surgery. Boost protein, lower carbs, and remove sugar from the dietplan.

• Two days before and the first week following surgery. Ingest only clear fluids which are caffeine- and - carbonation-free.

• For the Next three months. It's possible to add pureed food into your dietplan.

You will usually have the Ability to eat regular, Wholesome food about 1 month following your surgery. You might discover that you just eat less than prior to the process since you will get full fast and will not feel overly hungry.

Your restricted diet and smaller foods may cause some Nutritional deficiencies. It is important to compensate for this by choosing multivitamins, calcium supplements, a monthly B-12 shot, and many others as recommended by your physician.

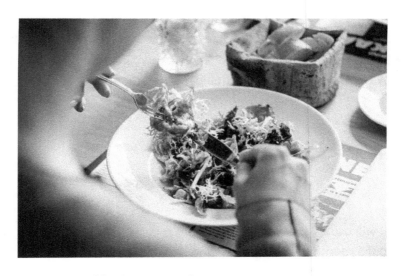

Is it covered by insurance?

In the USA, most health insurers realize that obesity is a risk factor for other health conditions that may result in serious medical issues. Because of this, many insurance businesses cover gastric sleeve surgery for those who have a qualifying state.

In accordance with the Centers of Medicare & Medicare Services (CMS), Medicare will cover gastric sleeve surgery if you meet the following requirements:

• Your BMI is 35 or greater

• You've one or more obesity-related health ailments

• You had been not able to eliminate the weight by simply modifying your diet and exercise habits or simply by taking drugs

Medicare does not cover gastric sleeve surgery in case you are Obese but do not possess an obesity-related health state.

Without health insurance policy, the price of gastric Sleeve surgery may vary widely from 1 area into another, and also from 1 centre to another in the exact same geographical location. Normally, the price could range from $15,000 to over $25,000.

Given this wide variation, it is Ideal to study and Speak to Several operative and surgeons facilities to find one you are comfortable with -- and also one which satisfies your budget.

The Main Point

Gastric sleeve surgery is one of several Kinds of bariatric Surgery choices. It works by making your stomach smaller so that you eat less. Since the dimensions of the gut are reduced, you will also realize that you are less hungry.

To be eligible for gastric sleeve surgery, you need to meet specific criteria. You have to show that you have attempted other weight-loss strategies -- such as diet, exercise, and weight loss medicines -- with no success. Other qualifying standards comprise your BMI and if you have some obesity-related wellness conditions.

Should you follow a healthy diet and exercise regimen frequently after gastric sleeve surgery, you could have the ability to shed more than 50 per cent of your extra fat within 24 weeks.

However, as with the Majority of surgical procedures, there's the danger of side effects and complications. If you are considering gastric sleeve surgery, speak to your physician about whether you are eligible for this process and if it is a secure solution for you.

Long-Term Infection after Gastric Sleeve Surgery

Gastric sleeve surgery, also called a sleeve gastrectomy, removes about 80 percent of their gut to promote weight reduction. Besides the dangers inherent with any surgery, gastric sleeve surgery could lead to a vast range of physical and psychological health issues. Those associated with weight and nourishment straight stem from how the staying, tube-like section of the stomach can only hold about 4 oz or 120 milliliters--a substantial reduction from its regular capability.[1]

Risks vs. Rewards

The remarkable decrease in belly size which results from Gastric sleeve surgery means you may only consume about half a cup at a time (at least initially). Since the quantity of food which may be consumed is limited, the amount calorie which may be obtained in is diminished. This is what contributes to weight reduction.

Gastric sleeve surgery is irreversible and May Lead to positive Health results for obese men and women who've fought with achieving and maintaining weight loss. And general, gastric sleeve is deemed secure when compared to other commonly performed surgeries.

Deaths from the procedure are rare, and if done by a qualified physician, the surgery has minimum complications. Nevertheless, when they do occur, complications may range from minor annoyances to important and possibly life-altering troubles.

Severe complications are those that occur shortly afterwards surgery. They include pain, bleeding, antastamotic flows (from the links between the intestines), and blood clots.2 the chronic issues detailed here are long-term, which means that they appear or persist six months following the onset of surgery.

Surgery is a tool, not a magic bullet. It requires you to follow release directions, limit food consumption, and adhere to the program supplied by your physician. It's likely to overeat and possess minimum weight reduction after surgery. It's also likely to have a severe complication either because of inadequate adherence for your post-surgical strategy or the surgery itself.

Gastric Sleeve vs. Bypass vs. Banding

There are various kinds of bariatric surgery, of which Gastric sleeve is merely one. There are lots of differences between these, and you need to examine each these options with your physician prior to deciding a process so you are able to guarantee that what you select would be the ideal alternative for you.

Listed below are two key long-term factors to keep in Head:

• A gastric sleeve is permanent. Contrary to the gastric band process --in which the ring that "cinches" the gut to split it into 2 components could be removed if There's a difficulty --that the portion of the gut eliminated with the sleeve process Can't Be substituted if there are issues or complications using digestion.

• You will not shed as much weight using a gastric sleeve. While individuals who have gastric bypass surgery generally shed weight and maintain a greater proportion of extra weight long term in comparison with people who have gastric sleeve surgery, skip can pose with it's own set of hard long-term troubles.

• Weight and Nutrition

• While the Goal of gastric sleeve surgery would be to encourage weight reduction, there's a possibility you can not shed as much as expected or that you shed weight, but get it back. What's more, while the decrease in food intake makes it possible to reduce calories, which also means that you're consuming fewer calories --that could cause deficiencies.

• Failure to eliminate

• That is a Serious problem in which the surgery is unsuccessful for weight reduction. The pouch might be too big, the individual may dismiss discharge directions, or a different issue could be found that prevents weight reduction.

• Regain

• From the First days following the surgery, the stomach pouch that remains is quite little and will hold approximately half a cup of food at the same time. With time, the pouch stretches and can accommodate larger quantities of food in a single sitting. This dilation allows bigger meals to be absorbed and may eventually lead to weight reduction weight or stopping reduction beginning

• Losing Weight after surgery simply to acquire all of back it normally starts in the next year following surgery, if it happens at all. Bariatric processes are a excellent tool for weight reduction, but if customs aren't altered and preserved, it's likely to acquire some or all the surplus weight again.

• Nutritional Shortfalls

• Unlike Many gastric bypass surgeries, patients that have a gastric sleeve process don't have any change in their capacity to consume nutrients in the gut. On the other hand, the remarkable drop in food intake may result in problems in taking in sufficient nourishment. Problems such as nausea and diarrhea may also lead to problems with consuming enough nutrients and calories too.

• In such Cases, a perfect whole-foods diet might not be sufficient to provide all the requirements of their human anatomy. Because malnutrition can be extremely severe, your physician may suggest using vitamin and mineral supplements, medicine, and other interventions to keep you long-term.6

- **Food Intolerance**

- One of The advantages of a gastric sleeve is the fact that all foods may be consumed after the process; other bariatric surgeries need you to avoid particular foods. But, that doesn't mean that the body will endure all kinds of foods.

- A 2018 Study discovered that food tolerance diminished after perpendicular sleeve gastrectomy, especially in regards to foods such as red meat, rice, pasta, and bread. The researchers noticed that this is probably because of the physiological and anatomical alterations in limiting the quantity of food that you can consume at the same time.7

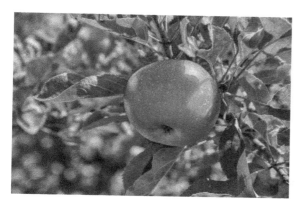

- **Physical Symptoms**

- Some Patients can experience gastrointestinal difficulties as a complication of gastric sleeve surgery. Although these may seem immediately after surgery, some patients might experience them for an elongated period of time. Sagging skin could be an additional complication which you experience after surgery.

- **Dyspepsia**

- Indigestion, Or an upset stomach, may be more regular following gastric sleeve surgery.8 this might be a result of the decreased volume of the gut and changes in how food goes through your gut and intestines.9

- **Nausea**

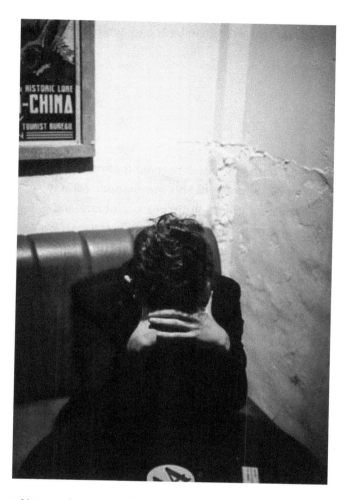

• Nausea is among the more prevalent issues that individuals face after sleeve gastrectomy.10 for many, this enhances after recovering from surgery, but for many others, the issue persists for weeks or long term.

• While it is not clear what causes nausea in this event, it can be partially as a result of food staying on your stomach for longer lengths of time.11 Nausea drugs can be found, which might be useful for many.

• **Diarrhea**

• For a few Patients, nausea is a severe issue that may persist following gastric sleeve surgery.12 This may happen for any range of reasons, such as alterations in gut microbiota and accelerated exposure to the small gut to undigested nutrients.13

• In instances Which last for an elongated period of time, the physician or even a gastroenterologist may have the ability to help stop nausea, which may result in malnutrition and dehydration.

• **Signs You Are Dehydrated**

• **Sagging Skin Care**

• This Complication is typical with all kinds of weight loss surgeries and can be caused by skin stretching throughout the time of obesity.14 A panniculectomy could possibly be an choice to get rid of extra skin, but many surgeons prefer to wait till the patient's weight has been steady for one or two years before removing extra skin.

- **Medical Problems**

- Gastric Sleeve surgery may cause medical conditions which range from moderate to severe. Speak to your physician if you have any worries about your probability of developing a health dilemma after surgery.

- **Persistence of Chronic Conditions**

- For a few, Eliminating chronic health problems--diabetes, hypertension, and many others --is your reason behind getting this surgery. Sometimes, these issues don't disappear after surgery, or else they might go away briefly from the first months or years following surgery and return afterwards.

- **Gastroesophageal Reflux Disease (GERD)**

- Heartburn, alongside other signs of GERD (bloating, feelings of fullness, and upset stomach), is common following this surgery and frequently requires medicine.5

- **Stomach Ulcers**

• Stomach Ulcers, called peptic ulcersare far somewhat more prevalent after gastric sleeve surgery And are generally diagnosed through an upper endoscopy following the patient Experiences bleeding (viewed as a dark, tarry feces or as blood in vomit) or pain In the gut region.

Gallstones

• Gallstones Are more prevalent following all kinds of bariatric surgery, building a cholecystectomy (surgery to remove the stomach) more prevalent to weight loss surgery patients.16

• Stomach Obstruction

• Scarring and narrowing of the outlet of the gut, also called stenosis, may make it hard or perhaps impossible to digest food. This complication is usually fixed by means of a physician that "stretches" or fixes the region which has been narrowed.

• Abdominal Adhesions

• The Organs and cells of the gut are obviously slippery, letting them slide past each other through movements like bending, twisting, and walking. After surgery, scarring may make these cells"stay" to each other. This induces a pulling sensation that can range from bothersome to debilitating with motion.Abdominal adhesions may also result in small bowel obstructions.

• Abscess

• An Abscess is a collection of infectious material (pus) that creates from the entire body in a pocket-like location. This typically happens shortly after the first surgery, because of spillage or leakage of intestinal contents. In the case of gastric sleeve surgery, abscesses have been diagnosed from the spleen, a few necessitating the manhood to be removed, but this Is Quite uncommon.

• Delayed Leak

• Most Suture line flows, also called suture line disruption or SLD, are found shortly after surgery. Sometimes, however, the region of the gut which was stitched together will start to flow months or years following surgery.

• These Later leaks are a lot milder but may be both annoying, and they might require drugs, hospitalization, or surgery to fix.

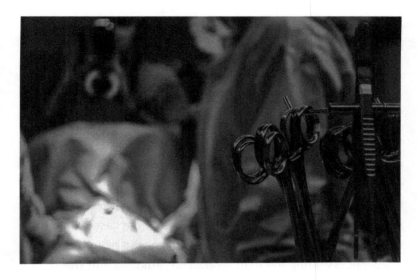

• Incisional Hernia

• A hernia can form at the website of any surgical incision. This danger is lessened by minimally invasive (laparoscopic) surgical methods, but a hernia may still form in the months and years after this type of process. Normally, that looks like a little bulge in the Website of a surgical incision.

• Psychological or Social Concerns

• Gastric Sleeve surgery can change your mental and psychological well-being, in addition to your relationships with other people. While weighing possible physical complications of this process is vital, these should not be overlooked.

• *Addiction Transfer*

• That is a Phenomenon that occurs to some people when they're not able to use food as a means to self-medicate their feelings. by way of instance, after a difficult day on the job, it's not feasible to go home and binge an whole container of ice cream--it simply won't match in the gut.

• Additional Kinds of addictions become more attractive since they're still possible using the smaller gut dimensions --alcohol misuse, drug abuse, and sexual dependency being one of the most frequent after surgery.

• **Divorce**

• From the United States, an average of 50 percent of marriages end in divorce; a few sources show that the speed of divorce following bariatric surgeries is as large as 80 percent.

• A 2018 Study indicated that divorce levels following gastric sleeve surgery might increase because the remarkable weight loss that impacts may impact the dynamics of a connection. This could occur if a spouse feels envious or no longer desired.

• Patients who are thinking of the surgery are advised to speak to their spouses about any possible problems and how they may handle anxieties should they appear.23 Couples might reap having this dialog with the assistance of a therapist.

• A Word by Very well

• One of The critical criteria that research scientists consider when assessing the success and security of operations is 10-year results. In cases like this, when it comes to the way patients maintain weight loss, what their general health resembles, and some other complications they've had because of surgery.

• It's Important to understand that gastric sleeve surgery is a fairly new process, so there's less 10-year information for gastric sleeve surgery than there is with other surgeries. Therefore, more long-term complications may be added to the listing later on.

Chapter 2 Recipes You Need in Your Bariatric Life

Traditionally we find ourselves at one of Both of These ships:

• Tasty, But wicked OR

- Healthy, But not yummy

Try our choice: Delicious and wholesome

Have your bariatric foods left you frustrated? The dietary Restriction that accompanies being a patient could be troublesome to put it gently. Imagine if you did not need to sacrifice the foods you like or your weight loss progress?

At it's most elementary level, weight reduction is a statistics game. If We're frequently in a calorie excess (consuming more calories than our bodies burn off) we get weight, if we consume fewer calories than we burn off we lose weight. It is actually that easy. Why is it so tough to drop weight on a constant basis?

Successful meal prep and portion control fix this Issue altogether. If you'd like guilt-free, flavorful and portion-controlled foods that work at any meal program you want to try out those recipes!

Get precisely the nourishment you want, in the serving Sizes you will need

1 thing which Makes cooking in bulk or one-pot recipes (such as at a crockpot or a casserole) hard for meal-planning is that the

amount of servings is not exact. Calculating the calories each serving necessitates busting a spreadsheet simply to receive your calories and macro amounts. Then you need to quantify out that quantity each time you get a serving. Not perfect.

Every recipe in this informative article yields individually packaged Single portions, making portion control as straightforward as it could be. It is possible to earn a whole batch and save the remainder for days and revel in stress-free, yummy meal-planning.

Chicken, Bacon and Ranch Wonton Cupcakes

This recipe brings All Your favorite tastes together in A tight, organized bundle. Who says you can not delight in the absolutely married taste of ranch and bacon when slimming down? Moderate ranch seasoning, bacon and lean chicken breast feeding make this an unbeatable alternative for healthier eating.

NUTRITION INFORMATION PER CUP:

152 calories | 10 g carbohydrates | 6 grams fat | 14 grams protein

INGREDIENTS

- 1 pounds uncooked boneless, skinless chicken breasts

- 1 Tbsp ranch seasoning

- two Tsp olive oil

- 5 pieces center-cut bacon, cooked crisp and chopped

- 3/4 cups Yogurt-based ranch dressing (like Bolthouse Farms)

- 24 wonton wrappers

- 4 ounces 2% shredded sharp cheddar

DIRECTIONS:

1. Preheat the oven to 375. Gently mist 12 cups at a normal muffin/cupcake tin with cooking spray and set aside.

2. Set the Raw chicken strips into a Ziploc bag and scatter with the ranch seasoning. Seal the bag and also shake/massage till the grain is coated with the seasoning.

3. Bring the Canola oil over moderate heat in a regular skillet. After the oil is hot, add the chicken pieces and stir them around to coat with oil. Arrange them into one layer and cook for 5-7 minutes, then turning sometimes, until the chicken pieces are cooked through. Remove the chicken to a cutting board and chop into small pieces.

4. Set the Chopped chicken into a mixing bowl and then stir in the chopped bacon and ranch dressing until well blended.

5. Push a Wonton wrapper to the base of all those coated cups in the muffin tin. With about half the chicken mixture, spoon evenly to the wonton wrappers. Sprinkle about half of the shredded cheddar evenly on the top of every cup. Press another wonton wrapper on top and repeat the layering steps together with the remaining chicken mixture and shredded cheddar.

6. Bake for 18-20 minutes before the wontons are golden brown and the materials are warmed through. Remove the muffin tin from the oven and allow cooling for 2-3 minutes before removing from the tin

Sesame Chicken Wonton Cups

If Asian fusion at a crispy package is not enough to get you Excited then we've got a bigger problem on our handson. Chicken does not need to be dull and dull. Do not overlook the sesame seeds along with the cilantro to actually make this 1 stand out! Makes 24 Wonton Cups.

NUTRITION INFORMATION PER CUPCAKE:

152 calories | 10 g carbohydrates | 6 grams fat | 14 grams protein

INGREDIENTS

- 8 oz boneless, skinless chicken breast

- cooking spray

- 24 wonton Wrappers, about 6 ounces.

- two tablespoons tahini

- two tablespoons soy sauce or tamari sauce

- two tablespoons maple syrup

- two tablespoons mayonnaise

- 1/2 cup thinly sliced snow peas

- 1/2 cup shredded carrot

- 1/2 cup thinly sliced scallions

- two Tsp chopped ginger and/or cilantro

- Black sesame seeds for garnish, optional

DIRECTIONS:

1. Place Chicken breast in a skillet and cover with cold tap water. Place over high heat and bring to a simmer. Reduce heat to keep a gentle simmer and cook till the chicken is no longer

pink at the middle and cooked through, 8 to 12 minutes, depending on the depth of the meat. Remove the chicken and let cool. Cut chicken into small cubes.

2. Meanwhile, preheat oven to 350°F. Coat two 12-cup mini-muffin tins with cooking spray. Cut off corners wonton wrappers to create an octagonal form. Gently press wrapper down into each cup. Lightly spritz wrappers with cooking spray.

3. Transfer the pans into the oven and bake till the wrappers have started to turn golden brown and so are crispy and simmer 10 to 14 minutes. Let cool completely.

4. Whisk Tahini, soy or tamari, maple syrup, and avocado in a medium bowl until smooth. Stir in the chicken and simmer until cold, 40 minutes to 1 hour.

5. Stir snow peas, carrots, scallions, and herbs into chicken mixture. Split the chicken salad one of wonton cups, about two litres tablespoons per day. Garnish with sesame seeds, if using. Drink immediately.

Meatloaf Muffin using Mashed Potato Frosting

While this can be another play around the cup-cake you have to give it the opportunity. If you prefer the basic principles of meatloaf and mashed potatoes you will enjoy every ideal snack of the healthful pairing. Use lean ground beef or turkey (at least 93% lean) and you're able to fit this to any diet. Makes 12 Cupcakes.

NUTRITION INFORMATION PER CUPCAKE:

120 calories | 12.25 g carbohydrates | 4.25 grams fat | 9 grams protein

INGREDIENTS

For your Meatloaf Cupcakes:

• 1.3 pounds 93% lean ground turkey

• 1 cup Grated zucchini, all moisture squeezed dry using a paper towel

• 2 tablespoon onion, minced

- 1/2 cup seasoned breadcrumbs

- 1/4 cup ketchup

- 1 egg

- 1 teaspoon kosher salt

For your Skinny Mashed Potato"Frosting":

- 1 pounds (about 2 medium) Yukon gold potatoes, peeled and cubed

- 2 big garlic cloves, peeled and halved

- 2 tablespoon fat-free sour cream

- 2 tablespoon Fat-free poultry broth

- 1 tablespoon skim milk

- 1/2 tablespoon Light butter

- Kosher Salt to taste

- Dash of Fresh ground pepper

- 2 tablespoon fresh thyme

DIRECTIONS:

1. Place the Garlic and celery in a large pot with salt and sufficient water to cover; contribute to a boil.

2. Cover and Decrease heat; simmer for 20 minutes or till potatoes are tender.

3. Drain and Pour onions and garlic into the pan. Add sour cream and remaining ingredients.

4. Employing a masher or blender, mash until smooth.

5. Season with pepper and salt to taste.

6. Meanwhile, preheat the oven to 350°.

7. Line a muffin tin with foil liners.

8. In a Large bowl, combine the turkey, zucchini, onion, breadcrumbs, ketchup, egg, and salt.

9. Place Meatloaf mixture into muffin tins, filling them to the surface, making certain they're flat in the top.

10. Bake Discovered for 18-20 minutes or till cooked through.

11. Eliminate Out of tins and put on a baking dish.

12. Pipe the "frosting" on the meatloaf cupcakes and function.

Chicken Broccoli Alfredo Wonton Cupcakes

If You want a healthy meal it generally will not contain Creamy Alfredo at any given capacity. Fortunately you are reading this recipe and will adore the way that it can fit into your diet if you're keeping your current weight or remain in your trip to your target weight. The Italian seasoning and light Alfredo sauce makes this feel like a cheat meal, you may return to the one many times! Makes 12 Cups.

NUTRITION INFORMATION PER CUP:

130 calories | 9 g carbohydrates | 5 grams fat | 13 grams protein

INGREDIENTS

• 1 1/2 Tsp olive oil

• 1 cup Broccoli florets, chopped little

• 2 cups cooked shredded or diced chicken breast

- 1 cup light Alfredo sauce

- 1/2 teaspoon Italian seasoning

- 1/8 Tsp black pepper

- 24 wonton wrappers

- 1 1/2 cup Shredded 2 percent Mozzarella cheese

- 1 Tbsp grated Parmesan cheese

DIRECTIONS:

1. Preheat the oven to 375. Gently mist 12 cups at a normal muffin/cupcake tin with cooking spray and set aside.

2. Pour the Oil to a skillet and deliver over moderate heat. Add the broccoli and cook for 5 minutes or until broccoli is tender, stirring occasionally.

3. Transfer the broccoli into a mixing bowl and blend with the chicken, alfredo sauce, Italian seasoning, and pepper. Stir until well blended.

4. Push a Wonton wrapper to the base of all those coated cups in the muffin tin. With about half the chicken mixture, spoon evenly to the wonton wrappers. Sprinkle about half of the Mozzarella cheese evenly on the top of every cup. Press another wonton wrapper on the top and repeat the layering steps together with the remaining chicken mixture and Mozzarella cheese. After finish, sprinkle 1/4 tsp of Parmesan cheese on the top of each wonton cup.

5. Bake for 18-20 minutes until golden brown.

Skinny Meatloaf Muffins with BBQ Sauce

This is just in time for summer! No need to kick the bbq For great when choices like these yummy muffins are from the cards. Applying lean turkey or ground beef makes it a no-brainer for your own health-conscious along with also the foodie alike. Do not skimp on the Worcestershire sauce and then experimentation with different bbq sauces! Makes 9 Servings.

NUTRITION INFORMATION PER CUP:

115 calories | 18 g carbohydrates | 2 grams fat | 18 grams protein

INGREDIENTS

- 1 bundle (~1.25 lbs) 99 percent fat-free ground turkey breast

- 1/2 cup bread crumbs

- 1 cup onions, finely diced

- 1 egg

- two tablespoons Worcestershire sauce

- 1/2 cup barbecue

- 1/4 Tsp salt

• Fresh Ground pepper, to taste

DIRECTIONS:

1. Preheat Oven to 350 degrees. Coat a routine (12-cup) muffin pan with cooking spray. Because this recipe makes 9 meatloaf muffins, you will just fill 9, not 12. Put aside.

2. To create Bread crumbs: 1 piece or multigrain bread. Set in a blender and pulse before made into crumbs.

3. In a Large bowladd ground turkey, bread crumbs, onions, egg, Worcestershire sauce, 1/2 cup barbecue sauce, salt, and pepper. With your hands or a large spoon, then thoroughly blend together until well mixed.

4. Insert Meatloaf mix to the 9 muffin cups, flattening out the shirts. Top each meatloaf muffin using 3/4 tbsp skillet and spread evenly on top.

5. Bake for 40 minutes. Run a knife around each muffin to loosen it in the pan. Remove to a serving plate.

Crunchy Taco Cups

Mexican food is usually packed with cream, cheese and unnecessary fats. These generally calorie dense choices cause blissful overeating. If you create these taco cups you will find the best of both worlds: flavorful, south-of-the-boarder flavor without the guilt which normally follows! We enjoy low sodium taco seasoning. It tastes just as nice and it is ideal to prevent excessive sodium once we can. If you're feeling "elaborate," substitute the Rotel tomatoes with a few freshly grated tomatoes. The tomatoes and thin coating of melted cheese makes this an instant classic. Makes 12 Taco Cups.

NUTRITION INFORMATION PER CUP:

178 calories | 10.4 g carbohydrates | 7.3 grams fat | 16.8 grams protein

INGREDIENTS

• 1 pounds lean Ground beef, browned and drained

- 1 Envelope (3 tbsp) taco seasoning

- 1 (10-oz) can Ro-Tel Diced Tomatoes and Green Chiles

- 11/2 cups Sharp cheddar cheese, shredded (or Mexican mix)

- 24 wonton wrappers

DIRECTIONS:

1. Preheat Oven to 375 degrees F. Generously coat a normal size muffin tin with non stick cooking spray.

2. Blend cooked beef, taco seasoning, and berries in a bowl and stir to blend. Line each cup of the prepared muffin tin using a wonton wrapper. Insert 1.5 tsp taco mixture. Top with 1 tablespoon of cheese. Press down and put in a second layer of the wonton wrapper, taco mix, and a last layer of cheese.

3. Bake in 375 for 11-13 minutes before cups are warmed through and edges are gold.

Chicken Cordon Bleu Wonton Cupcakes

Chicken Cordon Bleu can make you think about a standard feast Hall buffet, however, give this a try and you will have a change of heart. 1 thing which Chicken Cordon Blue has gotten is that the mixture of cheese and flavorful noodle paired with lean, healthful chicken. Those aspects are not lost here in this ideal "cupcake." Makes 12 "Cupcakes.

NUTRITION INFORMATION PER CUP:

152 calories | 10 g carbohydrates | 4 grams fat | 17 grams protein

INGREDIENTS

• 12 ounce (two 1/2 cups) cooked diced or shredded chicken breast feeding

• 3 ounce thinly sliced deli ham, sliced

• 8 wedges Of the Laughing Cow Light Swiss Cheese Wedges, sliced

- 1 teaspoon mustard

- 24 wonton wrappers

- 6 pieces 2 percent Swiss cheese, each cut into 4 equal pieces

- 0.75 ounce seasoned croutons, crushed

DIRECTIONS:

1. Preheat The oven to 375. Gently mist 12 cups at a normal muffin/cupcake tin with cooking spray and set aside.

2. In a Microwave-safe mixing bowl combine the ham, chicken, chopped cheese wedges, and mustard and stir together. Set the bowl in the microwave and heat on high for 1 1/2 minutes till contents are still warm. Use a spoon to mix contents and smush the cheese wedges till they have coated the beef.

3. Push a Wonton wrapper to the base of all those coated cups in the muffin tin. With about half the chicken mixture, spoon evenly to the wonton wrappers. Put one of the two% Swiss bits

on top of each cup. Press another wonton wrapper on the top and repeat the layering steps together with the remaining chicken mixture and 2% Swiss cheese.

4. Bake for 10 minutes and then remove it in the oven. Sprinkle crushed croutons evenly on top of each cup and then return the pan into the oven for another 8-10 minutes before the wontons are golden brown and the contents are warmed through.

Crab Salad at Crisp Wonton Cup

We Are in Need of variety in our diets, otherwise we get burnt out on Foods we might love and have loved for years! Chicken and steak are fantastic, but we want an offering from the sea to round out our diet. All these crab salad cups are exactly what you want if you are overlooking that flavor of the sea! Makes 18 "Cupcakes" (6 Servings) 1 Serving is 3 Cups!

NUTRITION INFORMATION PER CUP:

170 calories | 17 g carbohydrates | 7 grams fat | 9 grams protein

INGREDIENTS

For your Wonton Cups:

• Cooking spray

• 18 wonton wrappers

• two Tsp olive oil

• 1/4 Tsp salt

For the Dressing:

• 1 teaspoon lime zest

• two tablespoons fresh lime juice

• 1/4 Tsp salt

- 1/8 Tsp black pepper

- 1/2 teaspoon dried hot red pepper flakes

- two Tsp olive oil

For the Salad:

- 1/2 pound lump crabmeat

- 1 stalk Celery

- 1/2 cup finely diced mango

- 1/4 cup Thinly sliced scallions

- two tablespoons coarsely chopped fresh cilantro leaves

DIRECTIONS:

1. Preheat the oven to 375 degrees F. Spray two mini-muffin tins with cooking spray.

2. Brush the Wonton wrappers with acrylic, and then put each wrapper to a part of a mini-muffin tin. Gently press each wrapper to the tin and then arrange so that it creates a cup form. The wrapper will float itself and then stick up from this cup. Sprinkle with salt and bake for 8 to 10 minutes, until browned and crispy. Remove from the tin and permit wrappers to cool.

3. Meanwhile Whisk together the zest, lime juice, pepper, salt, and pepper flakes. Add the oil and whisk until well blended.

4. In a Medium bowl, toss together the crabmeat, cherry, celery, scallions, and cilantro. Add dressing and toss to blend. Fill each cup with all the crab salad and function.

Thai Chicken Salad Wonton Cups

Chicken salad could be as entertaining as waiting in the DMV, are we correct? Insert some Thai taste to this dull classic and you are really onto something. Chicken could be so versatile and that's evident in this yummy chicken salad cup. The wonton cup provides the essential pinch into the salad. The lime and citrus seeds actually provide this the different Thai taste you're certain to love. Makes 12 Cups.

NUTRITION INFORMATION PER CUP:

74 calories | 6.4 g carbohydrates | 2.4 grams fat | 6.2 grams protein

INGREDIENTS

• 12 wonton wrappers

Dressing:

• 1 garlic, smashed

• 11/2 tablespoon Lime juice

• 2 tsp rice vinegar

• Two 1/2 tsp Fish sauce

• 1 teaspoon soy Sauce

• 11/2 tablespoon Eucalyptus oil (or grapeseed, vegetable, or alternative neutral-flavored petroleum)

• 1 teaspoon sugar (or honey)

• 1 -- 2 Birds eye candy, deseeded and finely chopped (or 1 -- 2 teaspoon of chili paste or hot sauce)

Chicken Salad:

• 11/2 cups shredded cooked chicken

• 11/2 cups finely shredded cabbage

• 3/4 cup carrot, finely julienned

• 1/3 cup Finely chopped shallots/scallions

Garnish:

• Sesame seeds

• Fresh coriander/cilantro leaves

DIRECTIONS:

1. Preheat Oven to 160C/320F.

2. Place Wonton wrappers into a normal muffin tin, then molding it to the cups. Bake for 12 to 15 minutes, until crisp and pale golden brown. Remove from the oven and allow the cups cool from the muffin tin. Store in an airtight container until required (stays clear for as many as 3 times).

3. Blend Dressing ingredients in a jar and shake to blend. Put aside for at least 10 minutes to enable the flavors to infuse.

4. Blend Chicken Salad ingredients in a bowl and toss to blend.

5. To serve: Discard the garlic clove in the Dressing, and then chuck it via the Chicken Salad. Split the Chicken Salad between

cups. Garnish with sesame seeds and cilantro/coriander, if using. Drink immediately.

Buffalo Chicken Cups

Are Buffalo wings wholesome? Obviously they're not. Can we Take pleasure in the flavor of buffalo wings and lose weight? Obviously we could. This recipe carries lean chicken and yummy buffalo sauce to make a multitude of sinfully yummy flavors. These can be your new favourite over the conventional hot wings! If you are not a fan of blue cheese, then no issue. Just substitute a few drops of fat free ranch dressing and there you go." Makes 24 Cups.

NUTRITION INFORMATION PER CUP:

70 calories | 4.6 g carbohydrates | 2.7 grams fat | 6.5 grams protein

INGREDIENTS

• 2-3 boneless, skinless chicken breasts

- 2 Tbsp. Olive oil

- 1/2 tsp. smoked paprika

- 1/2 tsp. chili powder

- 24 wonton wrappers

- 1 Tbsp. Butter, melted

- 1/2 cup Hot hot sauce

- 1/2 cup Blue cheese crumbles

- 3 scallions, sliced thinly

DIRECTIONS:

1. Preheat Oven to 350F degrees.

2. Brush Chicken breasts with olive oil, and then sprinkle evenly with smoked paprika and chili powder. Put in a skillet and cook for 20-30 minutes, or until the heart is no longer pink and the juices run clean. Remove chicken and let cool, then shred.

3. Meanwhile, Match a wonton wrapper into each of 24 miniature baking cups, then pressing on the wrappers closely but firmly to the sides of the cups. (Be careful to maintain the corners of each wonton wrapper available; differently, you won't be able to fill them) Bake for 5 minutes until very lightly browned. Maintain wontons in baking cups.

4. In a medium-sized bowl, stir together the melted butter and hot sauce. Add the chicken and stir fry until well coated. Then fill each wonton cup using a tbsp or two of chicken, then top with a pinch of cheese. Return wonton cups oven and cook for an additional 5-10 minutes, or till cheese is soft and melty. Remove and top with chopped scallions, and serve hot. These are best served immediately.

Boom Bang-a-Bang Chicken Cups

Coronation Chicken is a Royal dish lin Good Brittain Generally consisting of cooked poultry meat using an easy curried mayonnaise dressing table. For how easy the recipe is it is kind of amusing how it made its way on the feast menu to the coronation of Queen Elizabeth II in 1953. Nonetheless, it's delicious albeit easy...

These person lettus cups reveal the original character of Coronation Chicken however in healthful single portions. Enjoy!

NUTRITION INFORMATION PER CUP:

176 calories | 6 gram carbohydrates | 10 grams fat | 16 grams protein

INGREDIENTS

• 100g smooth peanut butter

• 140g Full-fat coconut milk or natural yogurt blended with 2 tablespoons desiccated coconut

• 2 tsp Sweet chili sauce

• 2 tsp soy Sauce

• 2-3 Spring onions finely painted

• 3 cooked skinless chicken breasts, shredded

• Two Baby Gem lettuces, large leaves split

• 1/2 Cucumber halved lengthways, seeds scraped out with a tsp, cut into matchsticks

• toasted Sesame seeds, for instance

DIRECTIONS:

1. On your smallest pan, lightly warm peanut butter, yogurt, 3 tablespoons water, candy chili, and soy sauce until melted together into a smooth sauce. Set aside and allow cooling.

2. Mix the Spring onions and chicken to the sauce and season. Chill before the celebration. Maintain the lettuce leaves and cucumber under moist kitchen paper.

3. To build, Add a package of lemon to each lettuce leaf cup, and a spoonful of the chicken mix. Sprinkle with sesame seeds sit on a huge platter for all to dig. Or just serve a heap of lettuce leaves alongside bowls of chicken and pineapple.

Ancho Chile Ground Beef Tacos

Street tacos Are Typically fried in oil and comprise fatty Variations of meat with veggies sauteed in oils. This causes some seriously high fat (little) tacos that make you hungry and needing additional food. That is no good once you're limiting calories to weight reduction. Satiety and decent nourishment is the title of this sport.

This edition of beef tacos will assess each the boxes. The Usage of lean ground beef and seasonings for taste keeps the calorie count low as well as the taste high.

NUTRITION INFORMATION PER TACO (4 ounce) :

171 calories | 5 grams carbohydrates | 6 grams fat | 25 grams protein

INGREDIENTS

- 1 tablespoon. ancho chile powder

- 1/2 tbsp. cumin

- 1/2 tsp. smoked paprika

- 1/2 tbsp. oregano

- 1/2 tbsp. garlic powder

- 1/2 tbsp. onion powder

- 1/2 tsp. coriander

- 1/2 tsp. salt

- 1/2 tsp. pepper

- 1 pounds. 95% Lean ground beef

- 1/3 cup water

- 1/2 tbsp. cornstarch

DIRECTIONS:

1. Mix Collectively ancho chili powder, cumin, paprika, oregano, garlic powder, onion powder, coriander, salt, and pepper. This produces a tasty homemade taco seasoning.

2. Brown that the Beef (or turkey) at a skillet until cooked through. Drain any excess fat. If you prefer you can add veggies in this step you can -- diced onions, yellow and red peppers, drained and canned diced tomatoes, or diced zucchini are yummy. Beans are also a tasty addition.

3. Whisk collectively the water and cornstarch. Increase the pan together with the taco seasoning and bring to a simmer. Let simmer for 3-4 minutes until sauce thickens.

Garlic Lemon Shrimp Kabobs

Kabobs are the greatest single-serving food. You understand How much you put on the skewer and every skewer is its serving. It will not get much easier than that. Using lean foliage creates this recipe standout since its essentially pure protein and calculable.

Add them into a salad or eat them on their own -- either way, these can keep you on course together with your regular diet!

NUTRITION PER KABOB (6 ounce) :

189 calories | 2 gram carbohydrates | 7 grams fat | 31 grams protein

INGREDIENTS:

- 1.33 pounds shrimp, peeled and deveined

- Salt and pepper

- 2 tablespoon Butter, melted

- 1/4 cup freshly squeezed lemon juice

- 4 tsp garlic, minced

- 1 teaspoon Italian seasoning

- 2 tablespoon Parsley, sliced

DIRECTIONS:

1. Preheat the oven to 450 degrees or preheat the grill.

2. Insert the Butter into a small saucepan. When it melts, add the garlic, lemon juiceand curry. Cook for 2-3 minutes until garlic is fragrant.

3. Twist the fish on skewers. Season with pepper and salt. To cook in the oven, then put on a baking sheet, and cook for 5-6 minutes until pink and cooked through. To cook on the grill, put

right on the grill and cook for 2-3 minutes each side until opaque and cooked through.

4. When the Shrimp is cooked, brush together with the garlic butter mix and serve.

The Bottom Line:

While bariatric surgery isn't the "simple way" as a few people Think, you ought to be loving life! Enjoying life to the extreme entails enjoying calcium-rich food. The aim for life after bariatric surgery must be to boost your health, but also enjoying life.

Obviously, the life requires discipline and Dedication, therefore use these recipes to remain on your path to anew you" and steer clear of dull, tasteless food!

Immediate Post Bariatric Surgery Diet

IMMEDIATE POST BARIATRIC SURGERY DIET: FLUIDS

There are 3 basic stages of ingestion after weight-loss Surgery, irrespective of type. 'FLUIDS', the very first, is frequently regarded as the most difficult. Many come home from surgery, feeling somewhat uncomfortable, certainly exhausted, clutching their clinic guidelines then hover from the kitchen uncertain about what to eat or drink following.

What to do? First of All, follow your physician and Bariatric group's advice to the letter. Some surgeons will urge clear then complete fluids for only a couple of days after surgeryothers for as long as 4 months. This will be to minimise digestion, so reduce the creation of waste and ensure maximum recovery of your gastrointestinal system.

'CLEAR LIQUIDS', the kind you can see that will comfortably travel up a straw, are on the schedule. They ought to be sipped slowly rather than gulped. It's necessary to get enough of these to stay hydrated, which actually means you will nearly always have one in your side from the first days. It's necessary that a number of these are 'supplements' to offer you a bit of nourishment.

Listed below are some typical great choices and you'll find Favorites one of them. What exactly does taste strange to start with, frequently too sweet, therefore dilute with ice or water to get a more acceptable flavour and concentration. It needs to be stated that number helps, ring the changes frequently so that boredom does not set in. Though there's a limited choice that is for a reason. They'll maximise recovery and you need to just move onto another phase when informed and prepared to achieve that.

General guidelines are that you must target for 2.5 to 3.5 Litres every day. It'll be quite tough to make this happen initially but do attempt. Spread them out equally. Everybody has distinct fluid requirements; the very best method to check you're well hydrated will be to have a look at the color of the urine. If output is light, you're drinking enough. When it's dark e.g. straw-coloured or darker or when there's minimal urine, then you want to drink more.

The recommended fluid portion size at any given time is usually believed to be less than 200 ml. At the very early days that this may look to be an enormous volume! Each beverage can be best taken more than one hour apart.

NEVER HAVE FIZZY DRINKS.

Fantastic CHOICES OF CLEAR FLUIDS

• Water

• Tea -- Warm conventional, herbal or fruit teas

• Java -- Warm, ideally light-hearted

• 'no-added-sugar' Or'sugar-free' squashes and cordials

• Bovril, Marmite or Oxo'salty' beverages diluted well with warm water

• sugar-free ice lollies

• sugar-free Jelly, composed according to packet directions

• Chicken, Beef or vegetable bouillon/broth/consommé or soup

• a whey Protein isolate fruit beverage such as Syntrax Nectar, composed with water --excellent for obtaining protein in the first days

Along with A DAILY MULTI-VITAMIN AND CALCIUM SUPPLEMENT

It may Look like an age but you'll reasonably quickly then Proceed on the'FULL LIQUIDS' phase which offers a bit more variety and nutrition to your dietplan. This is a very important stage because it prepares your own surgically-altered gut for longer food. This phase again may last only a couple of days or a couple of weeks based on surgical opinion. Always follow your surgeon's time-line.

Full liquids are the Ones that are believed smooth and pourable. Mix and match them with clear fluids to get great hydration during the day. Taste and flavour might still be off skew but variety is the secret to moving sensibly through this point and preparing your body for another one. It will get better each day and good customs could be immediately established at this point to reap dividends after.

Fantastic CHOICES OF FULL LIQUIDS

• milk Skimmed, semi-skimmed, soya, almond and Flora Guru active

• Milky Chai kind tea -- lightly-spiced for extra flavour

• Unsweetened Plain yogurt or yogurt with no additional sugar and fruit pieces

- Eloquent Cream-style (although not large fat) soups

- Whey Protein isolates beverages, hot, cold or freezing composed with milk or water

- Whey Protein isolates powder blended with milk or water and made in a ice cream

- Mashed Curry blended with a little soup or broth until lean and soup-like

- diluted Fruit juice

- Tomato or V8 juice -- warm or chilled

- Oatly -- Oat-based milk beverage

- Rice Fantasy first milk

- Slimfast Shakes and sauces, though Slimfast might prove too high in sugar for many skip patients

• Home-made Smoothies (although not too thick) and also shop-bought ones e.g. Innocent Strawberry and Banana, diluted if necessary using water

• Cocoa (created with 4 gram powder along with 200 ml semi-skimmed milk)

• Smooth-type cup-a-soups

• Highlight/Options Hot chocolate beverages

• Home-made Vegetable, poultry or fish broth, pureed until smooth and simmer into a smooth gliding consistency (slowly increase the depth as you advance through this point to the upcoming tender or pureed food phase)

• Low-fat and low-sugar custards

• Very gently put egg custards

Moderate Term Post Bariatric Surgery Diet

MEDIUM TERM POST BARIATRIC SURGERY DIET: SOFT FOODS

If You Don't experience any Issues with the Phase 1 'Fluids' regime then you'll immediately move onto the next phase which comprises smooth, pureed, tender and crispy food, typically known as the 'SOFT FOOD' phase.

This stage is generally followed for approximately 2-6 weeks after Surgery, though again consistently follow your bariatric group's information on when to begin and when to proceed.

Start gradually and make sure first your food choices Are loose and soft -- first phase baby food feel is what you're aiming for this. Progress to foods which may be easily crushed with a fork or blended to some 'slurry' using milk, sauce or sauce. Do not be put off if something does not match...try it a couple of days later. Paradoxically a few days something goes down readily and the next time it does not. Learn how to listen to your own body and its own signs of gratification or angry.

You will still have to be aiming for at least 2 minutes of Liquids every day as well as those little 'foods'. Do not drink for 30 minutes before and 30 minutes afterwards and goal for 4-6 little 'meals' daily.

Eat slowly and the moments you're complete STOP EATING! Only one Extra tsp of food may send your own body into overload and there's not any nice way of stating this...what went down will return up or make you feel really uncomfortable! Recall that your new stomach pouch is simply about the size of an egg cup.

You may find it very suitable to suspend soft foods in ice Cube trays for this particular point. We discovered a stash of them, ready ahead of surgery, so beneficial in the forthcoming weeks. Foods in this type can be ready quickly for serving, variety is guaranteed as opposed to the constant round of this same-old and wastage is reduced to a minimal.

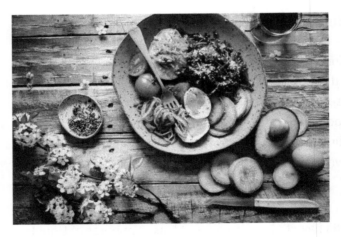

Listed below are some Fantastic food choices to your 'Soft Food' stage. Introduce these foods slowly replacing them since the days progress with ones which have more feel and flavour. Attempt to have 3 meals every day (ramekin or small tea plate dimensions).

Crispy foods, that will fall to pieces in water, for example Melba Toast, crispbreads, cream crackers and bread sticks may also be released from the latter times of Phase 2. Chew them completely before reduced to a smooth puree on your mouth. Do not confuse them for crispy foods e.g. salad and fruit that would cause difficulties at this point.

This is the point I think you Should Really Begin searching at preparing your recipes from scratch, so this way you understand just what's inside them. A lot of processed foods and prepared type foods have hidden fats and sugars to make them taste great but may be a banana skin to your weight loss surgery patient. Try out a few straightforward recipes to start with or be additional vigilant at ridding the trunk of pack nutrient advice of a food. You are aiming for low carb (as a rule than 3 percent fat i.e. less than 3 g per 100 gram recorded). In terms of sugar toleration levels fluctuate dramatically but I would not venture outside of the 6-7 gram struck per portion. It's believed that at levels past 10-15 gram you've got a strong probability of bypassing and sleeve 'dumping' syndrome and it will not assist those using a gastric group to maintain their calorie count reduced.

Fantastic CHOICES OF SOFT FOODS

• Weetabix, Porridge, Ready Brek having lots of skimmed or semi-skimmed

Milk to create a runny consistency

• mashed Banana with a small yogurt if enjoyed or using a low-carb and low-sugar custard

• Very soft cooked scrambled egg

• Finely Minced or grilled chicken or turkey in sauce

• pureed Fish at a thin sauce

• pureed canned fish e.g. tuna, pilchards, salmon or mackerel in a thin tomato

Sauce

• Soft and Smooth low-fat pate or distribute

• Plain Low-carb cottage cheese

• pureed Mashed potato and lean gravy

• pureed canned and extremely tender boiled vegetables like carrot and

Cauliflower

• Low-fat and low-sugar fromage frais

• Mild and Smooth low-carb and low-sugar mousse made with milk

• Heated Mashed potato mixed with grated low-fat cheese or low-fat lotion

Cheese

• milky Pudding like tapioca, sago or rice keep sugar into a minimum

• pureed Cauliflower cheese at a low-carb cheese sauce

• Pureed, Thickened or tender bit vegetable and poultry soups

• pureed casserole and stew dishes of a thinnish consistency

• Very Gently soft and cooked simple omelette

• poached Egg or even a soft-boiled one

• tender Beans, peas and lentils, pureed or simmer to get a small feel

• Thick fruit smoothies

• pureed Avocado

• Tiny Parts of home-cooked or ready-prepared and pureed main dishes

Like cottage pie, shepherd's pie, fish pie, fish-in-sauce, mild chilli con carne

Or their vegetarian choices created with quorn

• Low-sugar sorbets

• silken or smooth tofu

• crispy foods like crispbreads, Melba Toast, cream crackers and breadsticks

Long Term Post Bariatric Surgery Diet

Long-term POST BARIATRIC SURGERY DIET: THE FUTURE/FOOD FOR LIFE

Just when You're able to endure a Fantastic variety of foods From Phase 2, in the event you move tentatively onto Phase 3...ingestion FOOD FOR LIFE. Typically this happens between 8-16 weeks but everybody differs and constantly follow the recommendation of your very own bariatric team (and, simply since your dietician states you can eat grilled chicken, does not imply you can be able to do it straightaway, it sometimes requires a couple of times and retry events before you're ready to tolerate a specific food indefinitely). This is actually the point at which you ought to have the ability to attempt to consume an assortment of solid food, in tiny quantities. Consider with a side plate or kid's plate for a principle for serving size.

Foods to start with should possess a moist and soft feel so May need to be served with just a small sauce, cauliflower, sausage or dressing in order that they chew right into a moist mouthful, but as time goes onto a dryer texture is encouraged to get constriction and an perfect transition through the recently modified digestive system. These so-called 'slider' foods aid in the first days but may indicate that you're able to consume more in a subsequent stage only whenever you're searching to get 'satiety' and do not need foods to pass through the gut or pouch too fast. Gradually cut them down as you progress from week to week.

This is not a diet with a start and an end, nor is there Requirement to get a rush into the tape to reach a 'goal weight', take it gradually, learn to recognise when you're filled and satisfied and do not eat beyond there of satisfaction. As time goes on gastric bypass and sleeve patients may learn to Recognise this stage and gastric group patients will surely, over time, find their 'sweet spot'.

It makes Great sense to cook Foods for everyone in the Household Instead of different ones for everybody at this stage. Why be a servant to a different regime which will thankfully suit all? Everybody can benefit from the foods appropriate here, higher protein, low fat and reduced sugar. Insert an excess accompaniment for all those growing members of their family members or a candy treat from time to time to acquire a perfect equilibrium.

THE REGIME AND SOME RULES

HIGH PROTEIN, LOW FAT AND LOW SUGAR IS THE MANTRA

• Consistently Consume your PROTEIN FIRST (the beef, eggs, poultry, fish) in your plate, then proceed onto the veggies and fruit and eventually the carbohydrate part -- potatoes, rice, rice.

• Pick LEAN PROTEIN with almost any visible fat removed (e.g. chicken skin); target for LOW FAT (you won't always manage it again aim for under 3 grams fat per 100g); and consistently opt to get a minimal SUGAR edition of a meal or foodstuff (the syndrome called 'dumping' -- see page 00, is believed to happen when you consume between 7 and 15 grams sugar in 1 hit).

• Eat 3 Meals daily with two or three little snacks if needed. These should meet you. However beware of creating a 'grazing' eating routine of little snacks every day.

• Eat Wholesome, strong food. Soft food definitely slips down more readily but you may wind up eating more over the duration of daily. If your food is drier and stronger you'll normally consume less complete and stay fuller for longer.

• EAT SLOWLY and cease once you feel complete. Take miniature bites and chew every piece 10-25 times. CHEW, CHEW, CHEW AND CHEW more! As soon as you're feeling complete STOP! Gone are the times when you have to clean your plate.

• Maintain your Fluid ingestion. It's also a fantastic idea to not drink immediately prior to, during or after a meal so that your stomach is not complete from fluids. Get into this habit once possible of not carrying food and fluids collectively.

• Take your Multi-vitamin, calcium as well as some other supplement regular religiously... they will make certain you have the very best chance of obtaining all of the extra nutrition you need that might not be provided in the low amount of food you're eating.

• The Hardest nutritional supplement to stay on course with is unquestionably protein. Aim for 70 grams every day. Quite tough to start with and do contemplate a protein isolate powder in the event that you regularly fall short. A spoonful of the powder in food or as a beverage can easily and economically provide 25 gram or a third of your needs at one fell swoop!

CAUTIONARY FOODS

There are some cautionary solid foods, Which Might not be Tolerated in the long and short term. Proceed with care when ingesting them:

• Non-toasted Bread, particularly white and soft

• Over-cooked pasta and boiled rice

• Red meat using a fibrous feel like beef and chops

• Stringy Vegetables such as green beans

• sweetcorn, Lettuce and pineapple with a toughened texture

• Pips, Skins and seeds from vegetables and fruit

• Dried fruits

• No Caution, only a straight no to carbonated beverages and chewing gum (for life)

Conclusion

Gastric sleeve is a sort of bariatric surgery, also referred to as weight loss surgery. It's sometimes suggested for men and women that are extremely overweight, or who have health problems brought on by obesity. You should only consider gastric sleeve surgery after attempting choices. The very first step is typically to test modifications to your food consumption as well as your everyday exercise and activity. Additionally, there are some medications which could help people eliminate weight. Surgery is usually considered just after these other choices are tried. Slimming down after gastric sleeve surgery can help reduce issues with type two diabetes, diabetes episodes and blood pressure, also will help improve heart health. After the surgery, you are going to begin with liquid foods. During the upcoming few weeks you may change to pureed food, then to food. Your meals will be a lot smaller and you might need to quit drinking with meals because of your little stomach. You'll have to make substantial lifestyle changes following bariatric surgery to eliminate weight and keep it off. By way of instance, you are going to receive nutritional advice from a dietitian about the best way best to modify your eating habits to stay healthy while losing weight. Your foods will be a lot more compact than previously. And you're going to likely take vitamins or supplements for life. You'll also need to, and also be in a position to, raise the amount of physical activity that you do.

CPSIA information can be obtained
at www.ICGtesting.com
Printed in the USA
BVHW061947060221
599512BV00008B/1356